THE
JUST DIAGNOSED
GUIDE

SARCOIDOSIS

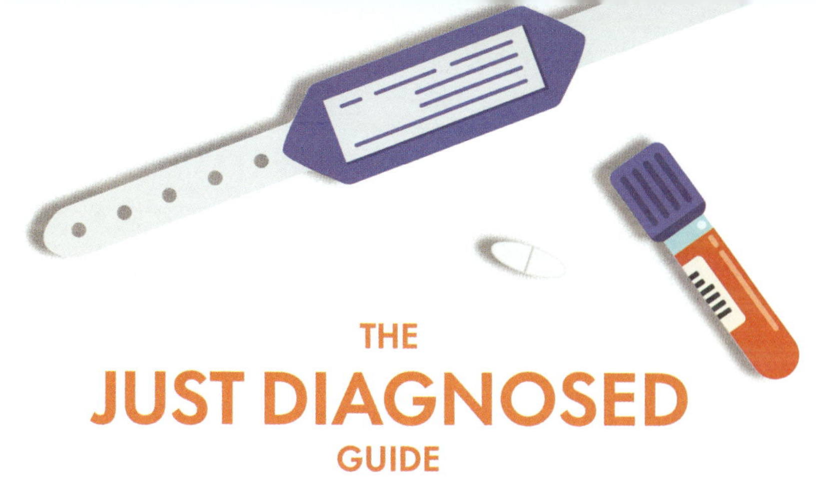

THE
JUST DIAGNOSED
GUIDE

SARCOIDOSIS

What You Need to Know Now (without Googling it)

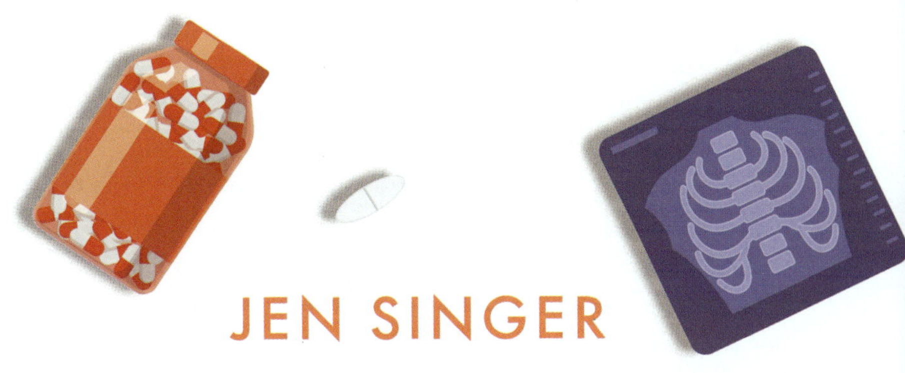

JEN SINGER

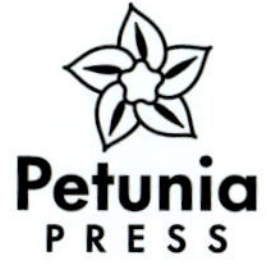

Petunia
PRESS

Red Bank, New Jersey

 Printed in the United States of America by Petunia Press, a division of MommaSaid, LLC, Red Bank, New Jersey.

Paperback ISBN: 979-8-9864391-9-8
Kindle ISBN: 979-8-9864391-5-0

DISCLAIMER:
FOR EDUCATIONAL AND INFORMATIONAL PURPOSES ONLY.

The author of this book is not a doctor, nurse, or any other type of medical professional. All content and information in this book are for informational and educational purposes only and do not constitute medical advice. The information provided is not a substitute for your doctor's care and does not attempt to diagnose, treat, prevent, or cure any physical, mental, or emotional condition. Please consult with your health care provider before taking any action or if you have any questions or concerns about your medical care, strategies, and options.

Contents

Just Diagnosed: Sarcoidosis

You've just been diagnosed with sarcoidosis and you have questions. You've probably never even heard of sarcoidosis before now, and you may feel confused and scared.

So you Google it.

Don't Google it.

I just Googled it for you to see what you might find, and I landed on a page where three doctors pontificated about the effects of sarcoidosis on quality of life as though they were talking about cars or goldfish, not people with feelings and families. Meanwhile over on the social media patient boards, a nervous patient asked what to expect from an invasive medical test, and the answers were on opposite spectrums of less-than-helpful: "Piece of cake!" and "Mine was HORRIBLE."

That's reason number one why you shouldn't Google your disease, at least not so soon after diagnosis. There's too much matter-of-fact medical information and a wide range of emotionally charged patient experiences that don't take into consideration your personal prognosis or your emotional state. Reason number two is that sarcoidosis is a rare condition that can affect various organs, and doctors differ on how to treat it, so it's easy to end up even more confused if you surf the Internet all willy-nilly.

I confess that when I was diagnosed with sarcoidosis, I did indeed Google it, but I had been a medical writer for top New York City hospitals, so I know how to navigate the information. I've researched everything from urinary tract infections to terminal brain cancer all in the name of work. But I've also researched some pretty big diagnoses of my own, including non-Hodgkin's lymphoma (remission since 2008) and heart failure (active, potentially caused by cardiac sarcoidosis). What I found was reams of information that could be frightening, confusing, or conflicting. Or all three.

I longed for empathic, curated, and filtered information, like the kind you get when you call a friend of a friend who's had the same diagnosis. I thought that kind of feedback belonged in a book that you can read shortly after a doctor tells you, "You have sarcoidosis."

This is one of those books, part of a "Just Diagnosed" series designed to help guide you through the turbulent time after diagnosis without scaring the heck out of you. It's not a substitute for your doctor's medical management or advice, but it will give you the basics of diagnosis, tests, medications, and living with and after sarcoidosis. Best of all, it will make you feel less alone.

Think of it as the knowing friend of a friend who has done the Googling so you don't have to.

Jen Singer

What is Sarcoidosis?

When you were diagnosed, you may have asked the question, "What the heck *is* sarcoidosis?" I had no idea what it was, and I had written about all sorts of other uncommon diseases and conditions as a medical writer.

Sarcoidosis is when tiny collections of errant cells, called granulomas, appear on any part of your body. It's most commonly found in the lungs and lymph nodes, but it can also affect the heart, eyes, skin, nervous system, and other organs. I was diagnosed with cardiac (heart) sarcoidosis, but I've also had sarcoidosis granulomas in my lungs and on lymph nodes.

Nobody knows for sure what causes sarcoidosis. Some believe it's the immune system's response to a virus, chemicals, or dust, and if that's true, I'm blaming Covid for triggering mine. I caught Covid early in the pandemic and the next thing I knew, I had a complete heart block, where the electrical system of the heart shuts down, which led to heart failure and a pacemaker. A heart failure specialist guessed that sarcoidosis was to blame and sent me for a cardiac PET scan, which he said confirmed his suspicions.

Symptoms can appear suddenly, like mine did, or take years to develop. It's typically difficult to diagnose as it is an uncommon condition that can look like other diseases, and doctors are trained to look for the most common causes of a chief complaint. It's that old medical saying, "If you hear hooves, assume it's horses." That's fine unless you're the zebra.

Some medical experts believe that certain people have a genetic predisposition to sarcoidosis that causes the body to react to an exposure by sending out a siren call to inflammatory cells. Picture it like an army that's assembled to fight the wrong war. Others liken it to an autoimmune disease, where the body responds to its own proteins by signaling inflammation. In other words, your body might be fighting itself.

Sarcoidosis is most common in people of African or northern European descent, people between the ages of 20 and 60, females, and those with a family history of the condition. If you're none of these things, consider yourself a unicorn among unicorns. Sometimes, it feels as though sarcoidosis just does its own thing.

According to the National Institutes of Health, about 60 percent of sarcoidosis cases resolve within two to five years, and relapse in these cases is thought to be low. For others, it's a chronic condition that can scar organs like the lungs and the heart, leading to long-term health issues.

Sarcoidosis can mimic a blood cancer called lymphoma, which is why some doctors might say, "At least it's not cancer." As someone who's had lymphoma, I concur that's a major plus, and the mortality rate for most types of sarcoidosis is very low. Huzzah. But that doesn't mean this condition is like a gentle summer breeze all the time, either. Neither are the treatments. (See Medications for Sarcoidosis.)

Left untreated, sarcoidosis can lead to lung infections, arrhythmias, kidney failure, glaucoma, or facial paralysis, depending on where the granulomas are located.

You can have sarcoidosis on more than one organ, so you may need more than one type of doctor to manage it. General symptoms of sarcoidosis include fatigue, weight loss, and painful and swollen joints or lymph nodes. Organ-specific symptoms include:

Lymph nodes: According to the Foundation for Sarcoidosis Research, 90 percent of people with sarcoidosis have lymph node involvement, causing swelling. The most common locations are the neck, armpit, and groin.

Lungs: Symptoms can include shortness of breath, chest pain, wheezing, and a persistent, dry cough. I've read that "pulmonary manifestations" are present in 90 percent of patients. In other words, chances are if it's in another organ, it's also in your lungs. It can lead to pulmonary fibrosis, which is scarring or a thickening and stiffening of lung tissue that makes it harder for the lungs to work properly.

Heart: Symptoms of cardiac sarcoidosis can include shortness of breath, chest pain, fainting, heart palpitations, and arrythmias, which are irregular heartbeats, swelling caused by fluid retention, and fatigue. You may wonder why a problem in the heart would lead to problems breathing. That's because blood that flows from the heart brings oxygen to the organs, including the lungs. Cardiac sarcoidosis may require treatments for arrhythmias and/or heart failure, including implantable cardioverter-defibrillators (ICDs), which are like circuit-breakers for the heart, providing a little jolt to get the heart's electrical system up and running again. I have one, and it provides peace of mind.

Skin: This type of sarcoidosis may cause a rash of red bumps that can be warm to the touch, sores on the cheeks, ears, and nose, hyperpigmentation (dark spots), and growths, particularly around tattoos or scars.

Eyes: Symptoms can include eye pain, burning and itchy eyes, redness, sensitivity to light, and blurred vision.

Nervous system (including brain and spinal cord): When sarcoidosis granulomas appear in the nervous system, they can cause weakness in the arms and legs; facial weakness; difficulty controlling walking, urination, or defecation; and in rare cases, paralysis.

Liver: Many people with sarcoidosis develop granulomas in the liver, yet most don't experience side effects. When they do, it can include fever, itchy skin, jaundice (yellowing skin and eyes), and a pain under the right side of the ribs.

How Sarcoidosis Can Affect an Organ

It's important to know where your sarcoid has set up shop, and to make sure you have the right specialist or team of specialists to handle your care. Sarcoidosis can lead to other conditions and complications, depending on the organ or organs it's affecting.

Lungs: This is the most common location for sarcoidosis, affecting some 90 percent of sarcoidosis patients. It can lead to pulmonary fibrosis, which is scarring of the lung tissue that makes it hard for oxygen to pass through the lungs and into the blood, and pulmonary hypertension, when scar tissue narrows or blocks arteries in the lungs, raising blood pressure. You will likely require a pulmonologist to oversee your treatment.

Pulmonary sarcoidosis has stages, but, unlike cancer, the stages don't signify a progression of the condition. Rather, they indicate where the granulomas are located. There are five stages of pulmonary sarcoidosis. In Stage 0, there's no sarcoidosis. You may wonder why there's a Stage 0, but it's because you can go into remission, which is an absence of symptoms, and that would be Stage 0. Stage 1 is when granulomas are on the lymph nodes only. In stage 2, they're also in the lungs. In stage 3, they're just in the lungs. In stage 4, they've caused scarring and damage to the lungs that's irreversible. The earlier the stage, the more likely the sarcoidosis will go into remission on its own.

Heart: Cardiac sarcoidosis affects anywhere from 10 to 25 percent of people with sarcoidosis. It can cause some potentially serious conditions, including: arrythmias; heart block, which is a blockage of electrical signals that regulate heart rate; heart attack; heart failure; sudden cardiac arrest; heart valve problems; and pericarditis, which is inflammation of the tissue sac that surrounds the heart. Depending on your diagnosis, you may require a cardiologist, heart failure expert, electrophysiologist (like an electrician for the heart), interventional cardiologist, and/ or a cardiac surgeon.

Brain and Nervous System: Though sarcoidosis typically affects the nervous system in just 15 percent of patients, it can cause some serious problems by blocking the nerves' ability to transmit between the brain and the body. Some of the conditions it can lead to include facial palsy, vision problems, muscle weakness, meningitis, hydrocephalus (fluid on the brain), and an underactive pituitary gland. You may need a neurologist and, if surgery is required, a neurosurgeon.

Eyes: Sarcoidosis can cause uveitis, an inflammation of a membrane in your eye, and glaucoma or cataracts. An ophthalmologist, who is trained in eye surgery, treats sarcoidosis of the eye. (Note that optometrists are like primary care doctors of the eye, performing eye exams and monitoring the eye for conditions like glaucoma.)

Bones and Muscles: Though uncommon, sarcoidosis can affect the bones, including joints, and the muscles. This can lead to arthritis and muscle weakness. Typically, a rheumatologist oversees this type of sarcoidosis.

Liver: It's actually pretty common for sarcoidosis to affect the liver, but it rarely causes symptoms. When it does, it may lead to liver enlargement or swelling and cirrhosis, which is scarring (called fibrosis) that causes permanent damage. It can also cause your spleen to enlarge or lead to anemia. A hepatologist or gastroenterologist may oversee this type of sarcoidosis.

Kidneys and Urinary Tract: Sarcoidosis can cause the body to overproduce vitamin D, which can cause the body to absorb too much calcium, leading to kidney stones, which really hurt. So check with your doctor if you're taking vitamin D supplements. A nephrologist or urologist might oversee this type of sarcoidosis.

Other: Sarcoidosis can cause sinusitis and enlarged salivary glands, which make the cheeks look swollen (though I don't know how you'd notice it if you're on steroids). An otolaryngologist or ear, nose, and throat (ENT) specialist may be involved in this type of sarcoidosis.

Sarcoidosis can affect one
or multiple systems of the body.

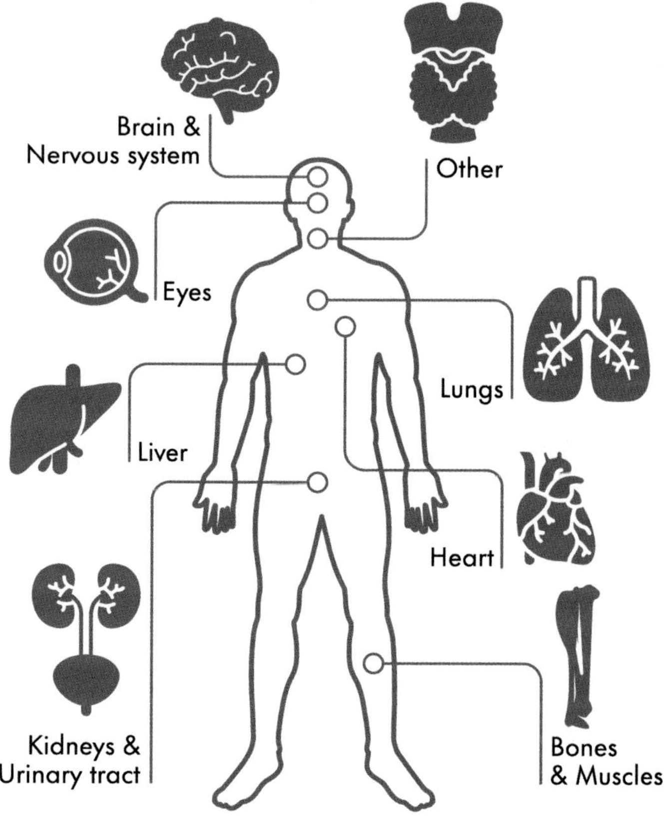

Diagnosing Sarcoidosis

Sarcoidosis can be difficult to diagnose. You may have a series of tests to confirm your diagnosis, assuming your health insurance plan* covers it. That's because other conditions, such as cat-scratch disease (brucellosis) and an autoimmune condition called Sjogren's syndrome, can mimic sarcoidosis. As a result, other conditions have to be ruled out as part of the diagnostic process.

Here's what you may expect:

Blood and urine tests: Your doctor may test for elevated levels of calcium, vitamin D, and inflammatory cells called angiotensin-converting enzymes (ACE). Note that elevated levels of these markers are just one piece of the diagnosis puzzle. Your doctor may also test for a low white blood cell count.

Your blood might also be tested to determine liver or kidney function. Sarcoidosis in these organs may not cause symptoms, and blood tests can help determine if the liver or kidneys are affected.

X-ray: While you can't diagnosis sarcoidosis with an X-ray alone, it can show inflamed lymph nodes or the presence of granulomas, which may indicate the need for other imaging tests.

PET/CT scan: Your doctor might order a PET scan or a CT scan or a combo PET/CT. A CT scan usually involves drinking a chalky substance called contrast or an injection of a contrast agent. The contrast helps make it easier for the doctor to see organs. In a PET scan, a radioactive tracer is injected into a vein to make it easier to see "metabolic activity," because fast-moving cells show up brighter on a PET scan. It seems to be the standard for diagnosing cardiac sarcoidosis though it's typically not considered as definitive as a biopsy, where the doctor takes a sample of tissue to examine under a microscope. (Taking a sample of cardiac tissue, though, is a little risky and does not always provide the answer either. As a result, the doctor may choose to order a pulmonary biopsy if sarcoidosis is present on the lungs.) CT scans might be used for pulmonary (lung) sarcoidosis, and sometimes a PET/CT scan is ordered.

Note: you'll have to fast up to 12 hours before these tests. The cardiac PET involves a very specific low-carbohydrate diet the day before the test. That's because healthy cells use glucose (sugar) as their main source of energy. Without sugar, they don't appear as bright as sarcoidosis. .

Bronchoscopy: In this test, a doctor checks out the lungs and air passages. Yes, you are sedated for this procedure. Why? Because a thin tube is passed through your nose or mouth and down your throat and into your lungs and who wants to be wide awake for that? Your doctor will look for granulomas and take a biopsy sample to examine under a microscope.

Mediastinal biopsy or Mediastinoscopy: The mediastinum is the area separating the lungs. These procedures are considered by some doctors as the only true way to confirm a pulmonary sarcoidosis diagnosis, but it comes with risks because it involves extracting a sample of tissue from the lymph nodes in the chest. You may wonder how your doctor gets the tissue. Most lung biopsies are performed with a lighted device called a mediastinoscopy, which is inserted into the chest above the breastbone or at the crease of the neck. Don't worry, you're not awake for it; you'll likely have general anesthesia. This procedure is used to rule out lymphoma as well.

Pulmonary function tests: These tests check how well your lungs are working. The most common test is spirometry, which measures air flow rate and determines the size of your lungs. You use a mouthpiece attached to a tube connected to a computer. Most medical websites will tell you that you'll "breathe in and out of the tube," making it seem as though you're just snorkeling. But no. You will likely have to suck in a bunch of air and then blow it out while someone says, "Keep going....keep going....okay, stop." It always makes me a little dizzy and then tired.

Cardiopulmonary stress test: This test checks how well your heart and lungs function during exercise. You may walk on a treadmill or ride on a stationary bicycle while attached to EKG equipment and an oxygen monitor. The speed, and for the treadmill, incline, rises at certain intervals. If you can't tolerate exercise, you may take a drug that simulates the effects of exercise on the heart.

MRI: This painless imaging test involves lying on a table while the machine around you loudly takes images of your insides. Doctors then check those images for sarcoidosis in the heart and nervous system.

Eye examination: An eye exam helps the doctor look for signs of sarcoidosis in the eyes. Your eye doctor dilates the pupils to view the back of the eyes, looking for signs of sarcoidosis. A biopsy might be performed.

Holter monitor: If cardiac sarcoidosis has led to arrhythmias (heart rhythm disorders or funky heartbeats), a Holter monitor can record the heart rate and rhythm. It's a portable, battery-operated device you wear around your neck, affixed to your skin, or on a belt loop for at least 24 hours to determine if you have irregular heart rhythms.

**I am writing the insurance information for those in the United States. Those of you in countries with universal healthcare can move along. Nothing to see here.*

Medications for Sarcoidosis

There's no cure for sarcoidosis, though sometimes it resolves on its own, and about a third of patients don't need any treatments. If your quality of life has taken a hit or the sarcoidosis could do serious damage because of where it's located, such as the lungs, heart, or nervous system, you'll likely get treatments and they can be, let's say, a bit tough.

Your doctor may prescribe immunosuppressants, which decrease inflammation in the body by weakening the immune system. If that sounds counter-intuitive, consider how sarcoidosis sets up shop in the body: It's an abnormal immune response that forms clumps of cells, called granulomas, on organs in the body. So the way to counteract this response is to suppress the immune system.

There are many kinds of immunosuppressants prescribed for sarcoidosis, all with the potential for various side effects. Take note: You may take these for months or even years until your sarcoidosis goes into remission or it doesn't and you have to switch meds.

Corticosteroids: Corticoid steroids are a type of immunosuppressant. This is usually the first line of therapy. We're mainly talking prednisone, which you may have taken in short stints for bronchitis or a nasty rash. You know, the blister pack with five pills on the first day, then four on the next day, etc.?

With sarcoidosis, though, you'll likely take high doses for a long time—months to years, depending on how well you tolerate it and your doctor's philosophy on medical management. There does not seem to be a standardized protocol for steroid treatments for sarcoidosis. My original cardiologist preferred to keep the steroids going for a year, while the next doctor believed in a six-month protocol.

I'm not going to sugar-coat it. Steroids can cause all sorts of nasty side effects, including cataracts, diabetes, glaucoma, hypertension, and osteoporosis. It tends to cause people to put on weight—I added 25 pounds, though lost most of it when I came off the meds—and the fluid retention can give you a roundish "moon face." Boy was mine full! Steroids can mess with your emotions, so if you find yourself inexplicably angry or weepy, it's probably the prednisone.

For me, the insomnia was rough, but it was also good for my career, because I'd get up at four a.m. to write. I was a bit hyper all day long, so I fixed the clothes dryer door, de-rusted my bicycle, painted the kitchen and my bedroom, and wrote a novel. Your mileage may vary.

Under my doctor's direction, I started on 40 mg a day and titrated (decreased the dosage) down by 5 mg each month—until I quit eight months into a year-long protocol because I just couldn't take the side effects anymore. That turned out to be just fine, as my sarcoidosis appeared to go into remission, nevertheless.

Of course this doesn't mean you'll get any or all of the side effects that I had, but you might get some of them, and it's best to know about them ahead of time so you can set your keep your expectations low.

If you have an allergic reaction, seek emergency medical help. That includes hives, sudden swelling in your tongue, throat or face, difficulty breathing, sudden blurred vision, or eye pain. There are alternatives to steroids, which I'll explain below.

Whether and when to call the doctor to report other side effects is always the question, because your doctor has a limited ability to fix it for you, short of taking you off or at least lowering the dosage of the steroids, and that presents its own issues for your prognosis.

Yet, if you experience pain, report it. I wound up in the ER with what one doctor suspected was a spinal fracture from weakened bones, which steroids can cause, but it was actually a particularly awful ulcer, courtesy of prednisone. After a visit to my gastroenterologist and some heavy-duty acid reflux medications, I felt way better.

Otherwise, I treated steroids like I treated chemo: It's something kind of rough that you have to endure in order to get healthy again, and it's going to go on for a long time. Hunker down. The good news? It's an old drug, so it's relatively cheap.

Off-Label Medications

The rest of the medications for sarcoidosis are "off-label," meaning they aren't FDA-approved for use in treating the condition. As a result, you may have difficulty getting coverage approval from your health insurance company. Your doctor may go to bat for you, writing a letter explaining why the medication is medically necessary for your condition.

Though they're not FDA-approved, many of these treatments are fairly common in managing sarcoidosis, and that can work in your favor. The reason for the push-back from the insurance company is because some of the meds are expensive. As a result, you could wind up footing a lot of the bill.

Some pharmaceutical companies offer discounts, either through coupons or patient assistance programs that provide free or discounted meds to low income or uninsured/underinsured people. For that, you'll have to apply. You can also check Medicaid for help, though their coverage may vary by state. I've seen patients covering anywhere from $0 to $750 a dose.

Methotrexate: It's a cell-killing agent used for treating cancer and rheumatoid arthritis. That's why if you Google it (though I told you not to), you'll see it's called a "chemotherapy agent." Don't let that flip you out. Most types of chemo are immunosuppressants, which is what you need to treat granulomas on the organs.

For sarcoidosis, it's often prescribed for months to years, most likely as an injection. It can affect the liver and kidneys, so it may require frequent blood tests. Some doctors recommend taking folic acid to minimize side effects, which can include nausea and fatigue. I've heard it can make your hair fall out as well; it *is* chemo. But it's not a common side effect and it typically doesn't make you go pool-cue bald like other chemos. (Been there, done that, saved on shampoo for a year.) Hair typically grows back once the medication is discontinued.

Remicade® or Humira®: If you can't tolerate prednisone or methotrexate or if those medications don't help dissipate granulomas, a doctor may prescribe Remicade® (infliximab) or Humira® (adalimumab), which are monoclonal antibody therapies for rheumatoid arthritis and Crohn's disease. Both are biologics, meaning they're made from living cells. These are so-called TNF-alpha inhibitors, which block the action of a protein involved in the body's inflammatory response. In other words, they reduce inflammation, and sarcoidosis is a clump of inflammatory cells.

These are expensive medications, with a single dose costing anywhere from $2,500 to $6,000 list price just for the medication, and more for the infusion in the hospital. As a result, it can take quite some time to get approval from your insurance company, if they approve payment coverage at all. Look for company coupons or patient assistance plans for help.

These medications are typically prescribed as an infusion that's performed in a doctor's office or hospital and administered with Benadryl®, which can make you sleepy. The infusions tend to take up to three hours, and patients have recommended bringing a snack, water, and even a blanket, but check with your doctor or the infusion nurse first. Note that some hospitals will help you get approvals for the supervised infusions, which can cost thousands of dollars a pop.

Side effects can include hypotension (lowered blood pressure) and fatigue. Some patients report feeling like they have a low-grade flu for hours or days after the infusions. It can be prescribed for months or years, and you may get infusions every four to eight weeks.

CellCept®: This is a drug to prevent organ rejection in transplant patients, but it's also used to treat sarcoidosis as an alternative to prednisone or when other medications fail to reduce or eliminate granulomas. It has not been tested in clinical trials for sarcoidosis, but it has been shown in small studies to make it possible for some patients with pulmonary sarcoidosis to reduce steroid dosages.

There is a lengthy list of potential side effects, ranging from hypertension (high blood pressure) to tachycardia (fast heart rate) to headaches. It can lower your white blood cell count and make you tired. Patients have reported nausea and heartburn, while others say it doesn't bother them at all.

Remember, it's an *organ-rejection drug*, so it's designed to keep your body from attacking and rejecting a transplanted organ. If that sounds scary, consider it's also one of the DMARDs—Disease Modifying Anti-Rheumatic Drugs—used to stop or slow the progression of rheumatoid arthritis. That means that thousands of people with RA have used it, so it's more common than it might sound.

It's also expensive. The pharmaceutical company that produces it offers a co-pay card program that appears to be offered regardless of income. You can enroll on their website. (Yes, you can Google that.) It covers "up to $10,000 per year," which means this is probably one pricey med.

Hydroxychloroquine: If your sarcoidosis affects the lungs or nervous system, you may be prescribed hydroxychloroquine, which came to fame during the Covid-19 pandemic. Prescribed to treat lupus, it's an anti-malarial medication that can decrease inflammation.

Its most common side effects are nausea, stomach cramps, vomiting, and headache. It can cause damage to the retina, resulting in blurred vision, seeing halos around lights, and night blindness, so you may need to have your eyes checked at least annually.

The good news is that this med is not (relatively) expensive. You can find coupons online. (Yep, Google that.)

Navigating Online Support Boards

Fewer than 200,000 people are diagnosed with sarcoidosis each year. Compare that to nearly 900,000 new heart failure patients or 1.4 million new cases of diabetes per year. So if you can find your sarcoidosis "people" online, it can make it easier to navigate treatments, doctors, and emotions. Hopefully.

Online, you'll find people who can answer your questions about medications, tests, procedures, and more. You'll meet fellow caregivers who are looking for information so they can best support their loved ones who are diagnosed with sarcoidosis.

You'll also meet unstable people. It is the Internet, after all. Worse, you can find a fair amount of misinformation and plenty of dismissive feedback, conflicting recommendations, or scary health stories. When your diagnosis is new, it's important to protect yourself from all that as much as possible, so approach support groups with caution.

Remember that everyone on these boards is dealing with their own trauma. Like you, they are patients or caregivers, and like you, they are seekers—of information, advice, opinions, empathy, and understanding. But their experience doesn't guarantee you'll have the same experience, especially with a condition that can affect so many different organs.

Other times, the boards are exactly where you need to be. It's worth it to join a general sarcoidosis support group and one specifically for your diagnosis, such as cardiac sarcoidosis. Search for your subject before posting a question because, chances are, someone else has already answered it.

The boards can be a great way to find out about new medications, new protocols, new procedures, and new philosophies of care. They'll also give you real-world experiences about side effects and procedures, plus day-to-day management. Who better to tell you what it's like to have a defibrillator implanted or what a pulmonary function test is like than someone, or several someones, who have been through it?

When you post, be prepared for someone to reply, "That's a question for your doctor." Every. Single. Time. That might be true, but one of the greatest assets the boards provide is information about what other doctors are doing. You'll have access to patients who are seeing some of the best sarcoidosis doctors in the country or in the world, including renowned practices at teaching hospitals. Their treatment will likely be cutting edge, and for a condition that's difficult to diagnose and to treat, the more information you have from top sources, the better. You might even decide to get a second opinion from one of those doctors if you aren't already a patient at such a practice.

You'll also find true support. Sometimes, you just need to know you're not alone in how you feel. People will cheer you on when you get good news or wish you well before a medical procedure or when you're feeling lousy and low. You might see a few photos of prednisone "full moon" faces and commiseration over drug prices, plus secrets on how to get discounts. There's something about getting support from people who are going through the same thing (and the people who love them) that's truly special.

When it comes to the sarcoidosis patient boards, love them or leave them, lurk or post, but they can at least make you feel less alone.

How to Work with Your Doctor's Office

When you have an uncommon condition like sarcoidosis that requires ongoing treatment, you will likely spend plenty of time in doctors' offices. How those offices run can affect your care and your wellbeing. Some will make you feel like a beloved guest and some will make you feel like a number, or worse, a nuisance. Between cancer and cardiac sarcoidosis, I've learned how to deal with all kinds of doctors' offices.

It's important not to confuse a doctor's office with any other business. They don't have to offer congenial service to keep the lights on, and there's usually a third party involved in their payments. While some of them are really quite wonderful, treating patients with respect and autonomy, others are not like that at all. Remember that they are often filled with overworked nurses and doctors who are weighed down by the demands of the U.S. healthcare system*. Still, that's no excuse for making you feel bad for asking a question.

I've had doctors who made me wait upwards of two hours for each appointment, nurses who sounded annoyed when I called for scan results, and billing departments that practically drowned me in paperwork. I've also had doctors who fought my insurance company of my behalf (and won), phlebotomists who managed to painlessly get blood from my chemo-wrecked veins, and nurses who held my hand while I cried because sometimes, you just need to.

No matter who your doctor is, make sure they have expertise in managing sarcoidosis. Ask how many sarcoidosis patients they've treated and how many they see each year. If you're in a rural or remote area, your choices may be limited, and I know of patients from all over the country who have travelled to see sarcoidosis experts at hospitals like the Cleveland Clinic and the Mayo Clinic for a second opinion. Of course, that takes resources that may be out of reach. Some insurance companies won't cover hospitals in other areas or states if there's an "expert" near you. That might mean that a pulmonologist or cardiologist in a strip mall near you lists sarcoidosis as a condition he treats, when in reality, he's had two patients—ever.

Here are some rules I've adopted when working with doctors' offices:

- **Use your contact wisely.** Make appointments, get prescription refills, report unbearable side effects, ask questions about diagnoses or tests that can't wait until your next appointment, and handle billing issues. Don't call or message with every little thought you have.
- **Use the portal.** If a doctor's office has a patient portal on their website, use it, but don't abuse it. It's a great place to ask questions between appointments, but not a great place for urgent needs, such as immediate

symptom relief or medication refills before your trip tomorrow. Most reply in 48 hours.

- **Write a script.** Remember, the nurses and staff who answer your call or read your message have to sort through what you're reporting to determine if you need an appointment, a new medication, a call back, or even a trip to the ER. Make their jobs easier and prepare a script to read on the phone or type into the portal that sticks to the facts. For instance:

> *I am a patient of Dr. [NAME]. My name is [NAME AND BIRTH DATE], and I am having a reaction to [NAME OF MEDICATION], prescribed on [DATE] to treat [SYMPTOM OR CONDITION]. My reaction is [BRIEFLY EXPLAIN REACTION]. I want to know if I can come off the medication and if there's an alternative that can be prescribed.*

- **Reel in the emotion.** When you call, try not to cry, though that sometimes comes in handy when you're trying to show the severity of a symptom. When steroids gave me a raging ulcer, a few tears were necessary to get across just how much pain I was in before anyone at my doctor's office took me seriously. That said, you don't want to get a reputation as that hysterical patient who calls in crying all the time.
- **Know your stuff.** The more well-versed you are about your sarcoidosis and its treatments, the more you help the doctor's office do their jobs. Keep a list of the medications and dosages handy, because sometimes

medical charts are not up to date. Learn the lingo, so that you know things like what a biopsy is, how to pronounce hydroxychloroquine, and your normal blood pressure rate.

What to Report When You Call the Doctor

Chances are, your symptoms and side effects from medications will vary over time. Ask your doctor for situations and side effects that should prompt a call to the office, especially when you are prescribed a new medication. Typically, that includes:

- A persistent cough you didn't have before
- Fatigue that persists
- Sudden, unexplained weight loss or gain
- A sudden, unexplained skin rash

If you're calling the doctor's office or using the portal to report a new symptom, here's a sample script:

> *"I am a patient of Dr. [NAME]. My name is [NAME AND BIRTH DATE], and I am having a new symptom of [SYMPTOM]. The doctor said to call if that happens. [REPORT RELATED NEWS HERE, AS IN "I STARTED ON XYZ MED LAST WEEK" OR "I HAD A PACEMAKER IMPLANTED TWO WEEKS AGO."] If I need to do something differently with my medication, please call me back at [PHONE NUMBER]."*

Making the Most of Your Doctors' Visits

Most medical web sites will give you the same advice for visiting your doctor:

- Write down your questions before your appointment.
- Bring an updated list of your medications.
- Bring someone who can take notes so you don't feel overwhelmed.

This is all good advice, and I'd add some more, especially when it comes to sarcoidosis.

- Keep a log of symptoms and side effects to share with your doctor. All too often, we forget just how difficult things have been or we're too afraid to share it with the doctor. If something hurts, say it hurts, not, "It kinda bothers me." Side effects and symptoms are not a moral failing on your part.
- Report even the most common or expected side effects of medications. Your doctor may dismiss it, saying something like, "Steroids do that." But you want it on your chart so that if it becomes unbearable, there's a record of your discomfort.
- If the side effects of a medication are causing major disruptions to your sleep, your work, your relationships, your exercise, you regular activities, or your mental well-being, tell your doctor. With sarcoid meds, there's a balance between toughing it out and being able to function day to day and sometimes, you can work out a different treatment plan or a lower dose with your doctor. Write yourself a script if you need one so you

don't back down when you see the doctor's white coat. (It happens. You're not alone.)

Choose Your Appointment Buddy Carefully

If you bring along a relative or friend to your doctors' appointments, choose wisely. A good health advocate is like a lawyer, reporter, and BFF rolled in one, but a bad one can interfere with your care and your wellbeing. Here are some qualities to look for:

- Listens well.
- Takes quality notes.
- Advocates for your concerns, not theirs. For instance, if they're squeamish about being awake for a procedure but you don't mind much zoning out on the Fentanyl (or whatever they give you) and watching the real-time X-rays of your arteries, then you don't need to spend much time talking about how to make you comfortable during the procedure.
- Doesn't hijack the appointment. (See above.)
- Makes sure your questions are answered.
- Makes sure you have what you need when you leave, such as a clear plan of action, any prescriptions, medication samples, a date and time for you next appointment, and paperwork for bloodwork, imaging tests, physical therapy, rehab, etc.

Getting Answers

While doctors typically serve as the appointment host, leading the conversation, don't let that role get in the way of your questions or concerns. Doctors are trained to ask a series of questions to determine your chief complaint, and yet sarcoidosis and its treatments frequently lead to multiple chief complaints. Each one deserves attention.

You may have shortness of breath that's worsened by exertion, but you're also going out of your mind on the steroids your doctor prescribed, and you'd like to know if you can lower the dose sooner than planned. This is no time to play down the side effects and promise to tough it out. If you have to, write down your concerns in big bold letters and only cross them off once your doctor has addressed them.

Doctor Visit Do's and Don'ts

Don't assume that what you report to the nurse at the start of the appointment will be relayed to the doctor. Tell them both. Some nurses work closely with the doctor while others simply take your vitals and move on to the next patient. If your doctor has a physician's assistant (PA) or nurse practitioner (NP) who meets with you first, take the opportunity to be as thorough as possible. The PA or NP's job is to sort through your information and present the key points to the doctor, and they typically have more time to spend with you.

Do ask your doctor what their concerns are during the appointment. For instance, if you report a new symptom, your doctor might furrow a brow and say nothing. If you ask what your doctor is thinking, it can lead to further discussion and discovery.

For instance, when an urgent care doctor was concerned about my symptoms that eventually landed me in the ER,

I had volunteered that I'd just flown to Washington State and my son had come home from New York City, both risk factors for contracting Covid in the early days of the pandemic. That led her to test me for Covid back when tests were in super short supply, and sure enough, it was positive.

Do make sure you leave with whatever the doctor promised, such as a prescription or medication samples.

Do get a second opinion. This can prove difficult with sarcoidosis because few doctors are experts in treating it. However, if you get a care plan from your local specialist, it may be worth it to make an appointment with sarcoidosis experts at a teaching hospital to make sure all your bases are covered. Post on sarcoidosis boards for names of renowned specialists or research them online. Or ask a nurse. They always know who's the best at what they do. Check how many medical papers the specialist has published, if they've spoken about sarcoidosis at medical conferences, and whether they've pioneered treatments. These are all signs of expertise. (These are all legitimate reasons to Google.)

Depending on your health insurance coverage (or lack thereof), it can be costly to go to such a doctor, but it can be worth it if you have a complicated case or you're not getting better with your current treatments. I left my doctor after he failed, even on appeal, to get an approval for a PET scan to determine if eight months of prednisone had reduced my sarcoidosis. My new doctor got the approval and the good news: no current organ involvement.

Do switch doctors if you think it will get you better care. Your health is more important than your doctor's ego. Be sure to get all your paperwork together before you leave. You may have to request your files and you may be charged. Nowadays, most information is in your patient portal. Keep hard copies of test results and doctors' notes just in case.

Making Your Medical Management Easier

You may feel like all you do is go to the doctor, get bloodwork, and take medical tests, especially if you're being treated by more than one type of doctor. Here are some ways I've made all that medical management easier:

Get a fax service: Some doctors' offices fax as though it's still 1999, so you might want to invest in a fax service that allows you to send scanned papers safely over the Internet or an old school fax machine, assuming you still have a landline to hook it up to. It's safer than emailing your personal medical records over the Internet.

Print and keep your own medical records. It's important to keep your own medical record files for several reasons. While many doctors' offices have converted to digital records that you can access via a patient portal, not all have, and it can cost money and take lots of time to get your records from a doctor's office. You may need them for a second opinion or if you switch doctors. Keep physical copies and scanned copies that you can fax or upload into a patient portal.

Add your primary care doctor to your paperwork. When you spend so much time at specialists' offices, your primary care doctor can get left out of the loop. Be sure to add your primary care doctor's contact information, including fax number, to your intake paperwork in any specialist's office. A good generalist can oversee all the plans made by various specialists, serving as a sort of stop-gap for your care. You may want to bring copies of your latest records to your primary care provider in case your specialists failed to send them.

Update your healthcare paperwork. Now is a good time to make sure that your will, living will, and healthcare proxy are up to date. You probably won't need them, but if you have a procedure that requires anesthesia, such as a biopsy or pacemaker implant, the hospital may ask for them. And if you don't have these documents, add that to your to-do list.

Keep your health insurance paid to date, and keep an updated list of your medications, doctor contact information, and emergency contacts in your wallet or purse, along with your health insurance card(s). If you have cardiac sarcoidosis, you may want to wear a Medical ID bracelet or necklace that includes information that EMTs or ER doctors may need to know, such as your diagnosis of arrhythmia or heart failure, or implanted devices like pacemakers.

Add your emergency contact information to your cell phone. Most cell phones include a location to add ICE (In Case of Emergency) numbers. Program them into your phone. You can also set up a Medical ID feature on your phone that first responders can check without your passcode. Check your Contacts or the Health app on your phone to add information such as your medical conditions, allergies, and blood type.

For the Caregivers

If you're a caregiver for someone with sarcoidosis, bless you. Also, thank you. Sarcoidosis is a rare condition that most people don't understand. As a result, the second-best thing you can do to support the patient is learn as much as you can about the condition and its treatments. The best thing? Never doubting how the patient feels.

Treatments for sarcoidosis are often no picnic, making the patient feel worse in order to get better, so a little empathy goes a long way. During the eight months I was on high doses of prednisone, I felt like I was awake more than I was asleep, and that's exhausting and made me feel a bit unhinged. I've heard that some meds make you what I call "Kryptonite tired," so sluggish and slow that it's hard to function. Others cause ulcers or cataracts, and some make the patient jumpy and quick to anger. And that's just the *treatments*. The condition also has its symptoms.

To be an effective caregiver, you will need patience and understanding. Treatments can last months or years while the patient waits to find out if they're even putting the sarcoidosis into remission, and sometimes they never achieve remission. This can feel like a long, lonely slog punctuated by doctors' visits, tests, and bloodwork. Understand that sarcoidosis can be a chronic condition that returns, even after extensive treatments.

If the sarcoidosis is extensive or if it's affecting a major organ, it can cause symptoms and complications that make it hard for patients to feel like themselves. That can include shortness of breath, fatigue, arrhythmias, fluid retention, itchy rashes, burning eyes, weakness in the arms or legs, and jaundice, a yellowing of the skin and eyes. Neurological symptoms can include confusion. For me, the doctor said the cardiac sarcoidosis caused a complete heart block—the electrical system in my heart was shutting down. Yet, I kept on working because it didn't feel "that bad" (and we didn't know it was my heart). Luckily, a friend persuaded me to call a doctor, who sent me to the ER.

Caregivers can serve as the wise voice of reason, a personal assistant/nurse/confidante rolled into one, or simply a ride to the doctor. A patient may need very little help but a lot of understanding, especially if you live together. Work out with the patient what role you can best play. Here's how you can offer to help:

- Find out the level of help the patient wants. Don't assume anything. Some patients prefer to handle as much as they can alone, while others would love it if you took over organizing and schlepping and filling up your nerdy binder with copies of medical paperwork, if that's your jam.
- Keep medical records, lists of medications, and contact information up to date.

- Be the eyes and ears for the patient. Take notes and ask questions at doctor visits.
- Join online sarcoidosis groups so that you can learn all you can from people in the trenches. There are also sarcoidosis support groups for patients with specific organs affected.
- Delegate tasks to family members, friends, and neighbors. You shouldn't have to do it all yourself.
- Listen. Sometimes, all patients need is an ear and some empathy. Don't try to cheerlead or tell them how to feel. Everybody just wants to be heard.

Managing Relapse

Remember, there's no cure for sarcoidosis, but you can have months or years without symptoms and it can disappear on its own for good. Sometimes sarcoidosis comes back, or "flares," typically within six months of stopping medications. This is also known as a relapse. The longer you are without symptoms—remission—the less likely sarcoidosis will flare.

If you dare to Google sarcoidosis, you'll find conflicting information about relapse rates. One study from Europe shows rates varying widely from 13 to 75 percent. But the Foundation for Sarcoidosis Research says that relapse is unlikely in patients who experience remission. It seems to depend on many factors, including the location of the sarcoidosis, age, race, and gender, making it hard to get more precise percentages on likelihood.

Even when you achieve remission, sarcoidosis can leave behind damage to organs. Patients with cardiac sarcoidosis may need a pacemaker with a defibrillator built in to prevent sudden cardiac arrest. I have one, and I'm grateful for the back-up system it provides. Damage to the lungs caused by sarcoidosis may require oxygen therapy, and neurosarcoidosis can require anti-seizure medications.

In rare cases, a patient may need an organ transplant, most likely of the lung, heart, or liver. But it really is rare, and sarcoidosis as a whole has a high survival rate.

Living with Sarcoidosis

Sarcoidosis can be a chronic health condition, and your experience and prognosis depend on which organ or organs it affects, comorbidities (other conditions you have which may be unrelated, such as cataracts or arrhythmias), access to healthcare, and other factors. You might battle shortness of breath while someone else's chief complaint might be a rash, and your battle might change over time.

You may find that how you feel varies day to day with ups and downs that can be disheartening at times. It's easy to think that one good day will lead to more, as though you heal in a straight upward line. But with sarcoidosis, it's never that linear. Take the good days while you can, and rest on the bad ones whenever possible.

Be prepared to change medications and dosages as your condition changes or if side effects become unbearable. One med might not work but the next one could be the key to remission.

There seems to be a misbelief that sarcoidosis doesn't hurt, but it can and don't let any doctor tell you otherwise. Still, don't assume that every ache is sarcoidosis; sometimes your toe is sore because you jammed it into the door, remember? But keep track of ongoing pain and fatigue and find ways to improve both. That can be through dietary changes to reduce inflammation in the body or via doctor-approved exercise, sticking to your medication protocol for the long haul, and finding ways to relax.

Consider psychotherapy or some sort of regular relaxation technique like meditation, peaceful walks, or my favorite, a float tank. This is a time to take care of yourself, even if it makes you feel selfish. There will be days when you feel like crap and others where you're almost normal. When it comes to sarcoidosis, it's often the meds that take the biggest toll on your body and your psyche.

The best advice for those of us with sarcoidosis comes from a Ukrainian tennis coach I once had. When the ball bounced where I didn't expect it to go, he'd yell across the net, "Adjust! Adjust!" Sarcoidosis requires us to adjust all the time, to how we're feeling that day, medication side effects, or what we can and can't get done because of symptoms. Adjust and keep on adjusting, and if all goes well, you'll have a good long remission.

Most of all, know you're not alone. There are plenty of us living with sarcoidosis, all doing the best we can. Be kind to your body and to your soul. You deserve it.